Unexplained Skin Problems
Home Treatment and Precautions

Don and Kellie Rainwater

ISBN: 1441443622

Unexplained Skin Problems

Many people in the world today have rashes, irritations, itches, and other types of skin problems that are unexplained. Even after a myriad of tests and other medical interventions they have constant or reoccurring skin problems that develop and can cause their life to be miserable. The most durable soul in the world can be brought to their knees when the itching and burning of their skin becomes unbearable and they can no longer maintain a normal lifestyle. Some of these skin problems leaves unsightly rashes, blemishes, and even scars which can cause embarrassment and social dysfunction. Even other skin afflictions can cause the sufferer to become reclusive and stay away from others because their constant itching draws attention to the in public.

Though many skin disorders have been cured in most cases, there is a growing list of skin problems are ones that elude patients, doctors, and other specialist while the sufferer still scratches and tries different remedies to ease the pain and discomfort. Problems such as shingles, hives, cold sores, ringworm, eczema, Staph infection, acne, boils, scabies, and Morgellon's disease haunt the patient with terrible itching and scratching. Though many of these have been explained, the traditional treatment or cure does not help people in certain situations.

For example, though diagnosed with eczema, one patient did not respond to any of the cures or treatments for the affliction and was cursed to spend her life scratching and itching the dry patches until she was forced psychologically to refrain to going out in public or seeking employment. Because of a skin disorder, this patient was economically, emotionally, and physically stricken to spend the rest of her life in isolation, poverty, and pain. She could not receive government assistance and without insurance, she had to suffer with this painful illness until she died at an early age.

Why do dermatologists not partition the government to list skin disorders, especially unexplained skin disorders as a disability? Most are not life threatening and are more a discomfort than a disability in the government and the medical communities eyes. With this attitude, there are millions of skin sufferers that will not find treatment within the medical community and will not receive disability in which many of the severe cases deserve. Most patients will have to look for non-conventional methods in which to ease their suffering which could help and in a few cases could be detrimental to the problem instead of helping it.

Shingles: Chicken Pox's Reemergence

Chicken pox is the virus that will later cause a person to suffer from shingles later in life. Most people think that once you have chicken pox the childhood disease goes away and you never have to worry about it again. Wrong! The virus stays in your system and never fully leaves your body. Certain catalysts like stress, cancer, chemotherapy, or aids, the virus are reactivated causing shingles. Happening to people over the age of 60 mostly, the virus has been known to affect more than 500,000 people annually and most of the times, the true origin, or cause of the outbreak is unknown.

The first symptom of shingles is unexplained pain or a sore sensation on one side of the body. The sensation is usually unexplained but the itching and constant ache is sometime unbearable. One or two days after the pain starts, red blisters, or puss filled bumps that are usually located near the pain and it will appear as a rash once the bumps are dried over with scabs. The scabs dry up and fall off after about twelve days and often there is a scar left. Most people who report the initial pain say that it comes in goes in spurts but the pain can be excruciating.

If you think you have shingles, do not scratch the scabs. This could cause a secondary bacterial infection. Most shingles requires some type of pain medication that helps the sufferer be alleviated from the pain and at the same time allows them to go about daily activities like their job or family life. There are medications that can be given to help reduce the time of the attack, but most home remedies include rubbing the infected area gently with warm soapy water and a clean cloth until the scabs dry up. This should be done several times a day to help the healing process begin.

Shingles is not contagious to someone who has had Chicken Pox, but if someone comes into contact with the puss filled sores and has not had the virus, they can contract Chicken pox. To prevent this, keep your rash area covered with a clean dressing. Remember, if you are a healthy person, shingles will not make you unhealthy, but just filled with pain. Some cases have been known to last for years. Pain management is about all you can do to get through the virus until it eventually goes away. If you are unhealthy or get sick a lot, check with your doctor because you may have an immune system deficiency that may cause the Shingles to appear more often.

Shingles: A Personal Story

A person very close to me was recently diagnosed with shingles. She began to have intense pain in her left breast, a pain that was unbearable. Many times she would have to leave work early because the pain became to extreme. The pain was a mystery until one day she noticed a small pimple on her back. It became apparent that every time the pain attack came, a small acne type of bump appeared on her back, neck, or head. Being a person who thought they could deal with pain, it took her several weeks to go to the doctor. Something anyone should have done as soon as something this severe began happening to their body.

Seeing a physician's assistant, my friend was diagnosed with shingles. She was given a medication that is usually associated to treat herpes. This and a pain medication helped her through the flair ups, but the bumps on her back still only came in a single entity and not in clusters as most shingles out breaks are. That and she was only 43 and most shingle episodes happen when a person is over sixty. The attacks came and went and still she would have attacks so bad that she could not function with daily activities. Not only quality of life but the embarrassment of not being able to deal with work and family began to toll on her.

One of the shingles precursors is stress. This lady just was promoted in a high stress job that put her on edge not only during work but after work also. The more stressful episodes that happened at work caused more pain to happen and the frequency of outbreaks increased. After a terrible bout she went back to the doctor. This time a real doctor, not a PA, reviewed her records and shook his head. He realized that she was misdiagnosed and was given a medication that not only relieved the pain, but relieved the anxiety that was associated with these types of outbreaks.

Since then my friend has been fine. The big mistake that the PA made is that the shingle sores are in a pattern along one strand of nerves. This cause pain in the tissue that is associated with that nerve cluster. If you have been diagnosed with shingles and you only have one bump that is present when pain is found, get a second opinion. My friend went through nights without sleep and missing days of work because of the misdiagnosis. Any skin problem or pain associated with a skin problem can be serious, so seek medical attention immediately.

Hives

If you have a red itchy area on your skin that are raised above the skin surface you may have hives. Hives can be a fraction of an inch wide or several inches. You can have hive in rings or in large patches. Hives can grow anywhere on your body whether it is an appendage, trunk of your body, or on your head and neck. People develop hives for one reason or another and it is estimated that fifteen percent of people in the world will develop some sort of hives during their lives. It is itchy and believe it or not, 80% of those reported cases have no explanation.

When you first get a rash of hives it may be a very alarming experience. The hives can fluctuate throughout the day disappearing at one time and then coming back full force the next. This can be very frustrating. You may wake up with hives all over your body and then by the time you get to the doctor, the whelps and rashes will have disappeared only to reappear when you get home. It is best to take a picture of the hives when they are active so that the doctor can get a full idea of what is going on with your body.

What causes hives? In the understood, explained hive episodes, doctors sa that haves are a result of histamine and other substances that are released from your cells and in all actuality a part of your skins normal processes. The hives are caused when the histamine is accidentally leaked into the blood vessels around your cells and enters the capillaries and blood vessels around the cell. Though common, hives can make the sufferer feel itchy, uncomfortable, and is damaging to the self esteem of the patient because of their unsightly appearance.

Most hives go away by themselves, but some require medical attention because it could be a sign of allergy or a immune disorder. The treatment of hives is usually the treatment of the symptoms and not the cause. Previously stated, the hives will go away most of the time on their own, but if you experience hives for the first time, visit your doctor and make sure that it is not something that is more serious. Hives can be treated with steroids, topical crèmes, and other medicines that will stop the itching while your body heals itself.

Hives: A Personal Account

An acquaintance had a terrible time with hives all her life. Once or twice a year the hives would appear in her skin all over her back, stomach, and sometime on the back of her neck. After going through a series of allergy tests with no results, the young lady accepted that she would have to suffer all her life. The hives were painful and unsightly and would appear when she was stressed or went to a new environment for vacation or business travel. Even a trip to Disney World was ruined because of these horrible outbreaks. Her life was miserable and she refrained from even going on vacation in fear of another hive attack.

Things that helped during the outbreaks were

hydrocortisone cream which eased the itchiness and the pain. The pain was so bad that even a cotton T-shirt could not stop the itch and discomfort, but the crème gave it some relief. Other methods that she used were to take a bath in a very small amount, a capful, of bleach. This should be monitored very closely because too much bleach can cause chemical burns. If the hives are on a child, this method should never be used. If done correctly, the bleach eased the itch and dried up the hives for a faster recovery.

The hives are thought to be caused, in this particular case, by humid conditions or a change in altitude. This particular lady grew up in Colorado and the hives, though they did break out at home, became more apparent when they visited tropical climates or climates that had a lot of humidity. There was no history of food allergy though scented detergents and fabric softeners sometimes caused irritation. To this one person, her skin problems were unexplained. She just treated symptoms, praying for a cure.

She told me that one thing that worked was a steroid shot. The shot was a cocktail of different things that seemed to work for about six months. She related that she went to Jamaica in March and did not have one single out break. Even though the climate was hot and humid, she got to enjoy a vacation for the first time in her life. The hives were gone and she even had a chance to get her first sun tan. Ask your doctor about the steroid cocktail if you have an unexplained out break of hives, it may be a blessing in a hypodermic needle.

Acne: The Scourge of the Teenagers Life

Almost everybody who is an adult has gone through acne. Though most of the time acne only affects teenagers and young adults, sometimes the red irritating skin rash can appear later in life. Acne is usually found in the oil-producing areas of the body such as the back, chest, in the face. Acne can also appear on your arms and neck if you are a person prone to oily skin. The bumps on your face and body may only last a short time but the psychological effects can go on for lifetime. The patient could experience a lack in self-confidence or self-esteem and even be socially withdrawn from the rest of the world. Acne can sometimes lead to depression.

Acne is caused by several different factors. The main cause is bacteria which live on your skin. This bacterium can create enzymes that dissolve the well in your skin in concert to be read in irritating. Male hormones called androgens are also a major cause of Acne. This hormone will lodge in the cell of the skin and in doing so, enlarges sebaceous glands in the skin. This acts as kind of a pump as the hormone creates more oil and at the same time does not give the oil a place to escape. That is why if you ever pinch a pimple, you will see that there is a lot of oil and puss coming from the Acne.

You can treat your acne without going to doctor. Just

make sure that you wash your face once or twice daily and remove all the excess oil. You can use just basic hand soap but you can always go to the drugstore and get some medicine or ointments to help clear up patches that are already infected. You can also get some cover up products that will cover the acne while it heals. Make sure you follow the directions on any over-the-counter treatment because if you don't, it can make your acne worse. Watch out for cosmetics and other cover-ups that are not medicated. They could make your acne breakout again.

When should you seek advice from a doctor? If your skin is beginning to feel tender and painful and the over-the-counter medications have not worked, it is time to seek professional help. If you are a woman and you are starting to see facial hair or see any irregularity in your menstrual cycle, you should seek medical advice quickly. Sometimes the acne will produce a fever and severe swelling; this is also a clue for you to visit your doctor and says you can. Acne can be a symptom of some larger disease or disorder so if you are any adult and have an outbreak of Acne it is time to see your physician.

Acne: A Personal Account of Shame and Pain

An acquaintance of mine, Susan was 15 years old. She was a happy freshman at a local high school. She had many friends and she had good grades. She was involved in many afterschool activities and was considered fairly popular by her peers. During the summer between her freshman and sophomore year Susan was afflicted with the teenagers curse, acne. It started out with just one or two small bumps on her forehead and a couple of small rashes on her jaw line. She took her mother's advice and tried to wash the areas every morning and every night with warm water, a washcloth, and hand soap. This helped a little but gradually the rashes and the pimples grew out of control.

When Susan as in her sophomore year most of Susan's face was covered with acne. Her forehead looked like raw meat from the irritating rashes and the bumps that accompany them. It hurt her to wash her face with a wash cloth, and over the counter medication stung her skin when they were applied. She didn't want to go to the doctor and wanted to try to heal the acne herself. Slowly Susan became ashamed of the way she looked and began to not take care of herself as well as she did before the acne arrived. Her self-esteem was low and she began to stay in the house with her parents and did not go out with her peers and friends anymore. Though the acne was bad on her face, the psychological and emotional damage the acne did to her personality was far worse.

Finally after going to doctor she was given antibiotics because the rashes and pimples have begun to get infected. She found out that bacteria has caused most of the rashes and that just by washing with soap and water, not all the bacteria were was washed off her skin. Instead she was festering a warm breeding ground for the bacteria which caused the acne to get worse and worse until it was finally painful and infected.

After following the doctor's advice, Susan began to clear her acne up around age 17. Her self-esteem was raised and she began to go out more. If you have acne that is not under control like Susan, you need to contact a physician immediately and see if your acne isn't caused by something other than bacteria or as a symptom of another disease or disorder. Though it is common for all teenagers to get acne, acne out of control can destroy not only the physical appearance of a person but it can also destroy their emotional self.

Cold Sores: Unpleasant for Everyone

Did you ever have an unexplained sore on your lip or around your mouth? This is commonly called a cold sores and are also known as a form of the herpes simplex virus type I. The virus can be spread from person to person by exchanging saliva by kissing or drinking out of the same container. If you have a blister type sore on your mouth, it is then that you are the most contagious. After the blister or sore has dried up and has a scab over it, you are then less contagious. It is untrue that you can catch cold sores from towels, washcloths, or other surfaces unless you come in direct contact with saliva during the infectious period.

Since the cold sores contain the herpes virus type I, then the sufferer should wash their hands as often as they should. If you have a cold soar you should share the same cup or can and you should not eat with the same utensils such as a fork or knife. If your cold sore is painful, you might want to try a cold compress to reduce the pain. That is about all you can do for home remedies. Studies have shown that most home remedies do not work and can actually cause the cold sore to stay around longer than it should.

You can try over the counter medications that are applied topically. Most of the products you find over the counter are usually for pain relief only and do not make the cold sore go away faster. Ibuprofen and Acetaminophen are also good to help relieve the pain and the itching associated with the cold sore. If the sun is a factor to your cold sore, then a sunscreen will not only protect the sore but will allow the sore to be protected while you are outside.

Two causing factors other than infection are stress and the sun. The best way to avoid a cold sore is to avoid the triggers of both. People are different and an out break of a cold sore is cause by different things. If you have cold sores often, keep a diary of what you have done or haven't done so you can pinpoint the trigger for your outbreak. If you have an unusually high number of outbreaks, contact your doctor and ask if there is a daily medication he or she can prescribe for you.

Ringworm: Not a Worm but a Fungus

Ringworm is not a worm but a fungus. The virus lives up to its name because it is elevated, red, and will make ring type sores on your skin. The center of the sore will not have any infection so it will look like a ring or circle. The sore, or the ring, may contain scabs or a crusty appearance while others might be filled with fluid or puss. Some of these sores can be about two inches across and may be itchy and painful. The sores will appear on the appendages of your body or on your face and neck. There is another type of ringworm that may appear on your scalp.

You catch ringworm by direct contact with animals or people who are infected. You can even catch the fungus from inanimate objects. A common way to catch ringworm is to step in infected fecal matter with your bare feet. You can even catch the fungus from exposure to soil that has been infected. If you think you are infected, there are several treatments you can use without going to the doctor. Sometimes the ringworm will go away on its own, but you can buy a topical cream that can be applied directly unto the lesions.

If you decide to use a topical cream, apply it on the sore itself and also on the skin an inch away of from the lesion and in the center of the lesion itself where there is no sore. Use the medication at least twice a day until the lesion disappears. Some over the counter medication that treats ringworm should include at least 2% miconazole and 1% clotrimazole. Brand names include Monistat, Micatin, Lotrimin, and Mycelex. Remember that ringworm is highly contagious so make sure you don't touch the lesions because it can spread and make sure you wash your body, hands, and clothes frequently to kill the fungus.

You need to seek professional advice if the ringworm does not respond to over the counter treatment. If they do not subside within one week of applying the medication, it is time to see your doctor. While you are treating your ringworm and you develop a fever or there is swelling in the skin or the infected appendage, it is time to get to the doctor fast. The swelling and fever could suggest that you have a bacterial infection within the sores and it needs to be treated as well.

Scabies: An Itchy Condition that is Contagious

Scabies is not a virus, bacteria, or a fungus. It is caused by a mite and it is a very contagious condition of the skin. The lifetime of the mites depends on the human host in which it uses as a food source. The mite cannot live on its own for more than thirty six hours without a human host, but with the human host it can survive a 12 month period. The mite will scratch into the human skin and lay eggs within the skin. As the eggs hatch they will grow into adult mites. People with scabies can have a condition that can make them suffer for weeks, months, or even years.

When you get scabies you will receive a rash that is very, very itchy, sometimes this rash is called the seven year itch. Sometimes the rash is not very big so scabies are hard to diagnose. The mite living in your skin can be passed on to other humans with close contact. Animals have a similar type of scabies but that type of mite cannot live on a human host. If an animal scabies mite lands on a human host it will die within three days. Scabies can affect anybody regardless of gender, religion, or socioeconomic status. It is most common between sexual partners. If you have a poor immune system you can get a higher form of scabies which will cause you to have scabs instead of just a minor rash.

There is no home cure for scabies and you will probably need a prescription from your doctor to get rid of the infestation. There are things you can do to prevent the spread of scabies to your family. You need to watch all your clothing, linen, and towels that you have used within the last three days of your outbreak. You must use hot water when you wash these things to kill the mites that live within the fabric. If you have other clothing around the house you think might be infected with the mites, put them in a plastic bag for about a week because the mites cannot live three days without its human host.

After getting back from the doctor and having a diagnosis of scabies, you may want to clean your house. You may need to vacuum your rugs or even have them shampooed. Anything you might have come in contact with you should be concerned that they are infested with scabies. Wash everything you have touched including stuffed toys, clothing, or any type of fabric such as the curtains or drapes.

Eczema or Dermatitis: Allergic Reactions Gone Awry.

If you have inflammation of the skin or an allergic condition that affects the skin, you may have eczema or dermatitis. Eczema is a lifetime condition for most people who have allergic tendencies. This type of skin disorder can be triggered by almost anything that comes in contact with the skin. Especially if the skin is sensitive, a dry, red, and inflamed area will cause intense burning and itching. Eczema is a common condition all genders, ages, races, and even can infect young babies. Most eczema cases begin early in life and it has been documented that 20% of all children are affected with this type of skin disorder.

For most people the disease will improve over time but others may have some form of the disorder all their life. Eczema is a very frustrating condition because not only are the rashes itchy, but they are very unsightly. If you scratch the rash it makes the condition worse and even medical treatment does not completely cure the condition. If you have never had an attack of eczema before you will notice that it will start with an intense itching. Later a rash will appear and the rash itself will become burning and begin to itch also.

You must refrain from scratching the rash once it appears. If the rash a scratched it may become crusty or ooze puss. Sometimes the rashes are just red bumps but they can also appear as a clear fluid filled bump. After these bumps dry painful cracks in the rash can appear. People have reported that the itching associated with eczema has been so intense that they have poor sleep. Eczema is often found near the face and can afflict the appendages of the body and the torso.

To help treat eczema or dermatitis you need to remove what is it ever is causing the allergic reaction in your environment. Some people have just changed laundry soap and the eczema has disappeared. If dry skin is the trigger, then the patient should take warm showers instead of a path. Remember when you take a shower make sure the water is warm and not hot. Hot water and soap causes the skin to dry and sets up a breeding ground for eczema to appear. If you are suffering from eczema you may want to not wear any cologne, under arm deodorant, or perfume that has a lot of fragrance. During an eczema attack it is also wise not to wear tight clothing or anything that will rub against the rash

The Heartbreak of Skin Tags

As you get older have you notice that it big mole and flaps of skin appear in weird areas of you body? These out-pouching of skin are called a skin tag. These little, benign, growths usually hangs from the skin where clothing usually touched the skin. Even places like your groin can be affected because the skin tags will appear even where there is skin to skin friction. You can also get skin tags on your neck, chest, and under your arm. If you are prone to skin tags, you will see them increase with age. Research has shown that there is a genetic link to skin tags and if your parents have them, there is a good possibility that you will have them also.

If you don't know what skin tags are, they are usually flesh colored but maybe will appear brown or lighter than the skin tone you have. They have either be smooth or wrinkled and can be tiny or the size of a dime. The skin tags usually hang on a stalk of skin and can be identified that way. Smaller skin tags will not have a stalk and will appear as bumps on the skin. If you twist the skin tag, the tag will become black or blue because it has lost its supply of blood. Sometimes bleeding will occur if you rub your skin tag with clothing or another surface. They are not painful and are a stand alone disorder, meaning they are not associated with other diseases or disorders.

You can treat your skin tags without even going to the doctor. Some people have used thread or dental floss to tie around the skin tag at its stalk. After a few days, the skin tag will naturally just fall off. If you don't want to do it your self, your doctor or nurse can remove your skin tags for you using a scalpel. There are no known medications to remove skin tags and it is advisable not to try wart removal on them. If the blade is not for you, you can ask your doctor to remove the skin tags with liquid nitrogen and freeze it off or have it burned off using electric cautery.

As stated before there is no medication that can cure skin tags and there is no medications that can help prevent them. If you had one skin tag, you are most likely to have more. Just find the method of removal that is right for you, and keep taking them off as they grow.

Morgellons Disease: A Medical Condition or Psychological

Morgellons disease is a controversial disorder that many doctors claim to be a psychological condition rather than a medical one. The disease has symptoms of crawling sensations on and in the skin and also disfiguring sores. Although the disease is not considered a medical condition by the medical industry, the Center for Disease Control is taking the matter seriously and has called Morgellons disease 'an unexplained skin condition.'

There are several symptoms to the disorder staring with skin lesions which will cause the sufferer intense itching or even pain in some circumstances. The patient will witness fibers that are in or on the lesions. These fibers can be white, red, or black. The sufferer will experience a crawling sensation on the skin that has be compared to bugs moving underneath the skin that feels like they are biting or stinging. The patient will become fatigued and will experience joint and muscle pain. Short term memory will be affected and there are even reports of behavior changes to the person infected. Other symptoms include a change in skin color or texture, stomach pain, and changes in vision.

There has been numerous reports of Morgellon Disease that began in the year 1674. Sir Thomas Browne, an English doctor, used the term Morgellons Disease after he witnessed small fibers coming out of lesions of a small boy. Since then, in the United States, there have been several hundred cases reported mainly in the states of Florida, California, and Texas. Even though so many people have reported the disorder, many in the medical community simply ignores their cry for help telling them it is all in their head.

Since Morgellons disease is not officially recognized, there are ways to manage your treatment on your own and with the right people. First, you need to gather a caring health care team around you that believes in the disorder. This will be hard because even if a doctor believes you, they will be embarrassed to admit it to their colleagues. You have to be very patient. If the doctor carries the visit to a diagnosis, you will be assured that you will receive the most up to date, peer reviewed treatment possible

While you are waiting and worrying, keep an open mind and do some research on the disease your self. You will be amazed to find that there are some brilliant minds out there working on a cure if not the treatments to the symptoms. If your Morgellons is causing other disorders like depression, seek treatment for those conditions.

The Heartbreak of Psoriasis

Psoriasis is another unexplained skin problem. It is usually the result of an inflammatory disorder that is usually chronic. There is sometimes a rapid multiplication of skin cells found in the epidermal layer. It is most commonly found on the head near the scalp, but can also affect the knees, feet, hands, and elbows. The genitals can also become inflamed. More than 4.5 million adults have psoriasis and many have the condition and do not know it. As stated, the exact cause is unknown, but there are guesses of genetic predisposition and factors that occur in the environment. Even the immune system is a major trigger, but what triggers the outbreak is still a mystery to science.

If you think you might have psoriasis, you may notice pink or red areas that seem to be thick, raised, or may just be dry skin. This is most common on the scalp, knees, and elbows or anywhere the skin is pulled tight around a bone or joint. The psoriasis can come in different forms. It could be as simple as a red areas or it could appear as flattened bumps. Some are accompanied by flaking skin and a dry ashy area. To treat your psoriasis, there are many over the counter drugs that can help. There are several lotions, creams, and lotions that have been known to be effective and when not, a small steroid shot to the affected area seems to work.

If you are treating your psoriasis yourself, you may find that whatever over the counter medication you are using might quit working. This is common because the skin cells get used to the change when you put that medication on. You might want to try a rotational approach to treating your psoriasis. Many dermatologists use this method. The idea is to change your psoriasis treatment ever two years. This not only gives the skin a chance to heal with the new medication but it will also take away the chance of side effects from the older medication.

Light therapy, or phototherapy have been known to work for psoriasis in many occasions. You can buy prescribed home light therapy kits, but natural sunlight in controlled exposure have been known to clear them up. Otherwise keep your affected areas away from sunlight outside the prescribed therapy time. Remember, there is no cure, but you can treat the symptoms yourself without going to the doctor.

Rosacea: Not Just an Embarrassed Look, but a Skin Condition

A skin disease that is not only embarrassing, it makes you look embarrassed all the time is Rosacea. Rosacea is a skin disorder that causes pimples and redness on your forehead, chin, and cheeks. When it is at its height in an outbreak it looks like adult acne. Sometimes the outbreaks are so severe it causes soreness and itchiness to the eyelids and eyes. If you live Rosacea untreated it can get worse and cause you not only to feel uncomfortable, but look uncomfortable. Rosacea can be treated at home, but for severe cases, visit your doctor.

Rosacea is a unexplained skin problem that tends to attack people who blush easily or have lighter skin. The problem is believed to run in families and is genetic. A myth about Rosacea is that it is a result of alcohol abuse. This is not true, but alcohol may make the outbreaks to seem more severe. The triggers of this skin disorder are not understood, but they are believed to be caused by several factors. Stress, hot baths, hot weather, and exposure to extreme weather can all be factors. To find your trigger, you might want to keep a diary of flare ups so you can pin down what the trigger is for you.

The symptoms of Rosacea usually appear to have a flushed face like they have just exercised or come in from the cold. The bumps appear around the nose, mouth, cheeks, and forehead. Sometimes tiny veins will appear on the infected areas that look like spider webs or varicose veins. The face will be very sensitive and any application of lotions, creams, or ointments will leave a stinging sensation on the patient's face. The eyes may become irritated and they will be void of moisture and feel dry.

There is no cure for Rosacea, but doctors can prescribe medications to treat the symptoms. Some suggest antibiotic pills or crèmes. Other physicians prescribe stronger medicines like Accutane and Retin-A. If you have advanced Rosacea, then surgery can be performed to at least bring back a un-tortured appearance. You can treat the symptoms yourself using over the counter medications. It is wise to seek the advice of your doctor for diagnoses and then try to treat your self unless the Rosacea becomes worse. As with all unexplained skin problems, get a diagnosis and then seek to treat the symptoms. The cure is not there but at least your health and self esteem will be maintained.

Ehlers-Danlos Syndrome Explained

There are a group of similar disorders called the Ehler-Danlos syndromes. With these syndromes you can bruise easily, skin that stretches too easily, and a weakness of the skin tissues. These syndromes are genetic and are usually inherited from the parents. The syndromes are categorized by which type of genetic accordance that has happened and which symptoms are displayed. Most of the syndromes have the symptom of a protein that is abnormal, the protein that acts as glue between the cells of the skin. Researchers have discovered that tenascin, a protein that is linked to the disorders, can play a large part in how the distribution of collagen in the tissues in the body that deal with connectivity.

Ehlers-Danlos syndromes are usually diagnosed through the history of the family tree and through clinical findings. Usually the doctor will take a skin biopsy to see what the chemical make up of the patient's skin is to make a final diagnosis. The syndrome acts individually so the treatment is as individual as the patient themselves. The most critical thing if you are diagnosed with these syndromes is skin protection. The patient most be wary of situations in which the skin will get scratched or punctured and they even have to watch out for the sun. If a wound occurs, prevention of infection is paramount.

If a wound occurs where the patient needs to be sutured, it would be very difficult to do so because the skin is so elastic. Along with the skin, injury to the joints must be avoided. Sometimes the patient needs to brace a joint so it does not fly out of place. If the patient exercises to build up muscle around the joint, then the joint will have a better opportunity to stay in place. People with these syndromes should avoid contact sports or any activity that would create injury.

Patients with Ehlers-Danlos syndromes have to live a different life than most other skin sufferers. It is almost like they are hemophiliacs because of the caution they must take when doing everyday activities. Something as simple as stepping on a nail or cutting themselves on the hand can lead to larger medical issues. The skin is so elastic medical personnel would have a hard time mending the skin with conventional methods. If you have been diagnosed with one of these disorders, please follow your doctor's advice, be careful, and let no cut, scratch, or puncture go unattended.

All advice in this book is given trough a novice's viewpoint. The material is presented from research in latest articles and peer reviewed literature. Your doctor's advice is the best course if you have any of these skin disorders.

www.ingramcontent.com/pod-product-compliance
Lightning Source LLC
Chambersburg PA
CBHW051421170526
45165CB00004BA/1909